Vegan Keto Delicacies

Low-Carb Cooking Recipes for a Balanced Lifestyle

Meadow Lambert

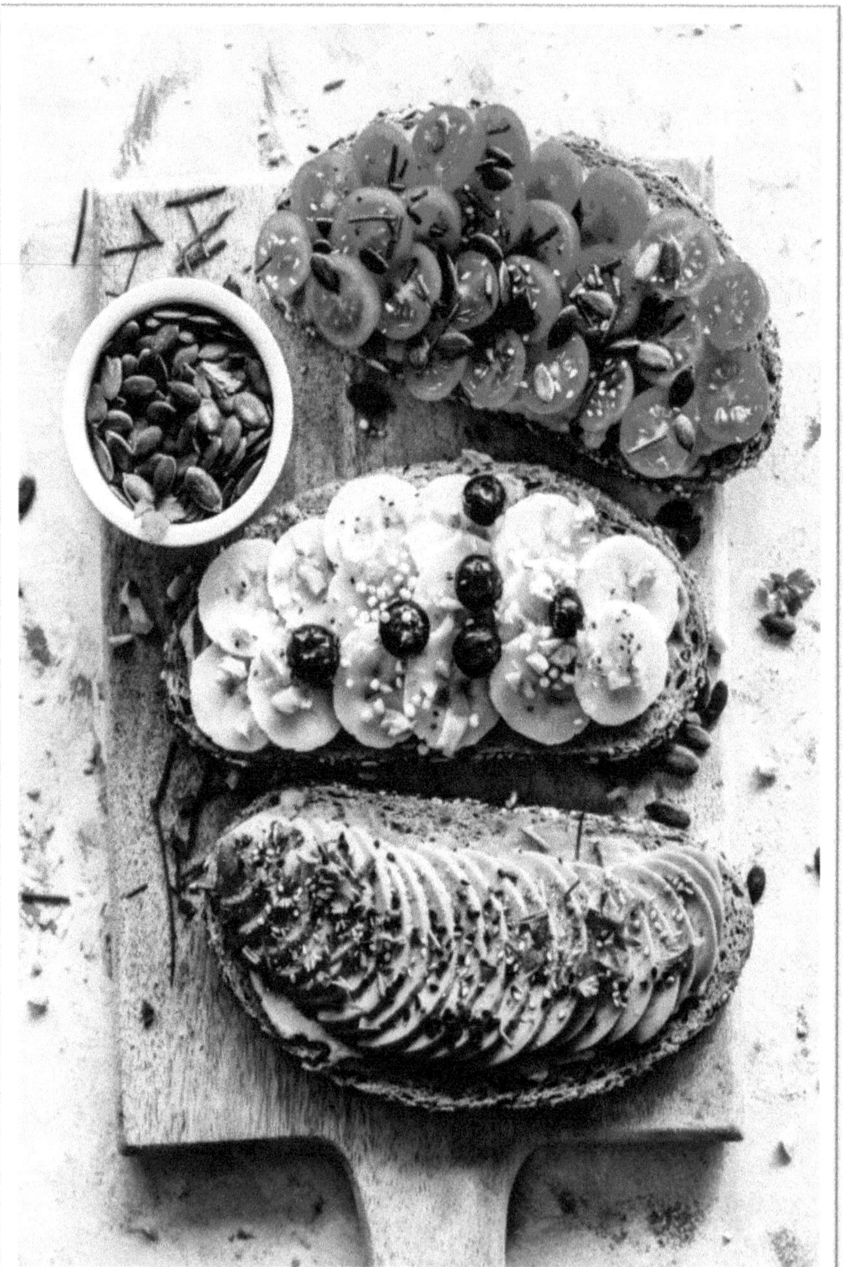

by reading this document, the reader agrees that under no circumstances is the author responsible for any losses, direct or indirect, which are incurred as a result of the use of information contained within this document, including, but not limited to, — errors, omissions, or inaccuracies.

Table of Contents

Beet and Clementine Protein Smoothie

Preparation Time: 10 minutes

Cooking Time: 0 minutes

Servings: 3

Ingredients:

- 1 small beet, peeled and chopped

- 1 clementine, peeled and broken into segments

- ½ ripe banana

- ½ cup raspberries

- 1 tablespoon chia seeds

- 2 tablespoons almond butter

- ¼ teaspoon vanilla extract

- 1 cup unsweetened almond milk

- 1/8 teaspoon fine sea salt, optional

Directions:

1. Combine all the ingredients in a food processor, then pulse on high for 2 minutes or until glossy and creamy.

2. Refrigerate for an hour and serve chilled.

Nutrition: Calories: 526 Fat: 25.4g Carbs: 61.9g Fiber: 17.3g Protein: 20.6g

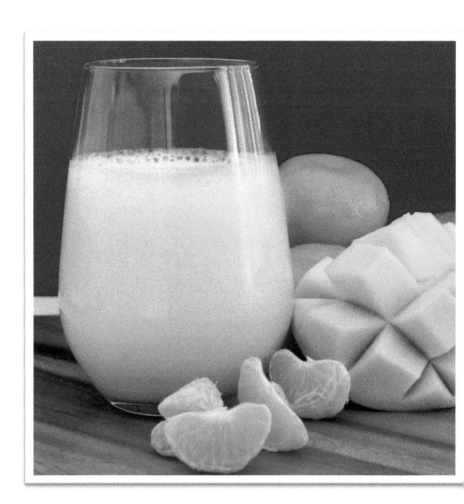

Italian "Meatball" Subs

Preparation Time: 5 minutes

Cooking Time: 55 minutes

Servings: 4

Ingredients:

- Chickpeas, liquid drained, rinsed – 15 ounces (1.5 cups)

- Bread crumbs - .25 cup

- Flaxseed, ground – 1.5 tablespoons

- Water, warm – .25 cup

- Nutritional yeast – 2 tablespoons

- Italian seasoning - .5 teaspoon

- Sea salt - .5 teaspoon

- Garlic powder – 2 teaspoons

- Sub rolls, medium – 3

- Vegan mozzarella cheese, shredded (such as Daiya or homemade) – .75 cup

- Marinara sauce – 1 cup

Directions:

1. Preheat your large oven to a temperature of Fahrenheit four-hundred and twenty-five degrees. Meanwhile, assemble your chickpea "meatballs."

2. In a medium-sized bowl for the purpose of mixing whisk together the warm water and flaxseed until all of the clumps are gone. Allow it to sit for five minutes.

3. Meanwhile, place the chickpeas in the food processor with the standard blade and pulse them until they are finely ground with no whole beans remaining. Place the chickpea meal into the bowl with the flaxseed mixture.

4. Add the sea salt, bread crumbs, Italian seasoning, nutritional yeast, and garlic powder to the chickpea and flaxseed bowl, combining the ingredients together completely with a spoon.

5. Using a mini cookie scoop or tablespoon measure out evenly sized "meatballs" with the mixture, rolling them into balls in the palms of your hands. Place these prepared meatballs on a baking sheet lined with kitchen parchment and allow them to cook in the hot oven for fifteen minutes before turning the pan around and cooking for an additional fifteen minutes.

6. Reduce the oven temperature to that of Fahrenheit four-hundred degrees.

7. Place the cooked meatballs in a large saucepan and add in the marinara sauce, heating it on a stove burner set to medium-low heat until the sauce is hot all the way through. Occasionally stir the chickpea meatballs in the marinara sauce so that they are evenly coated.

8. Fill the sub rolls with the meatballs and sauce, top them with the dairy-free cheese, and place them in the hot often on the baking sheet for fifteen minutes, or until the dairy-free cheese is melted and the bread is warm. Enjoy the subs hot and fresh from the oven.

Nutrition: Number of Calories in Individual **Servings:** 376 Protein Grams: 16 Fat Grams: 9 Total Carbohydrates Grams: 57 Net Carbohydrates Grams: 67

Chickpea Scramble Bowl

Preparation Time: 10 Minutes

Cooking Time: 10 Minutes

Servings: Makes 2 Bowl

Ingredients:

- ¼ of 1 Onion, diced

- 15 oz. Chickpeas

- 2 Garlic cloves, minced

- ½ tsp. Turmeric

- ½ tsp. Black Pepper

- ½ tsp. Extra Virgin Olive Oil

- ½ tsp. Salt

Directions:

1. Begin by placing the chickpeas in a large bowl along with a bit of water.

2. Soak for few minutes and then mash the chickpeas lightly with a fork while leaving some of them in the whole form.

3. Next, spoon in the turmeric, pepper, and salt to the bowl. Mix well.

4. Then, heat oil in a medium-sized skillet over medium-high heat.

5. Once the oil becomes hot, stir in the onions.

6. Sauté the onions for 3 to 4 minutes or until softened.

7. Then, add the garlic and cook for further 1 minute or until aromatic.

8. After that, stir in the mashed chickpeas. Cook for another 4 minutes or until thickened.

9. Serve along with micro greens. Place the greens at the bottom, followed by the scramble, and top it with cilantro or parsley.

Nutrition: Calories: 801Kcal Proteins: 41.5g Carbohydrates: 131.6g Fat: 14.7g

Matcha Limeade

Preparation Time: 10 minutes

Cooking Time: 0 minutes

Servings: 4

Ingredients:

- 2 tablespoons matcha powder

- ¼ cup raw agave syrup

- 3 cups water, divided

- 1 cup fresh lime juice

- 3 tablespoons chia seeds

Directions:

1. Lightly simmer the matcha, agave syrup, and 1 cup of water in a saucepan over medium heat. Keep stirring until no matcha lumps.

2. Pour the matcha mixture in a large glass, then add the remaining ingredients and stir to mix well.

3. Refrigerate for at least an hour before serving.

Nutrition: Calories: 152 Fat: 4.5g Carbs: 26.8g Fiber: 5.3g Protein: 3.7g

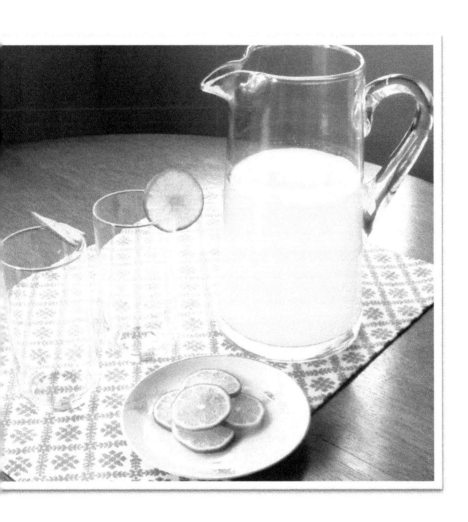

Curd Bread

Preparation Time: 4 hours

Cooking Time: 15 minutes

Servings: 12

Ingredients:

- ¾ cup lukewarm water

- 2/3 cups wheat bread machine flour

- ¾ cup cottage cheese

- Tablespoon softened butter

- Tablespoon white sugar

- 1½ teaspoon sea salt

- 1½ Tablespoon sesame seeds

- Tablespoon dried onions

- 1¼ teaspoon bread machine yeast

Directions:

1. Place all the dry and liquid ingredients in the pan and follow the instructions for your bread machine.

2. Pay particular attention to measuring the ingredients. Use a measuring cup, measuring spoon, and kitchen scales to do so.

3. Set the baking program to BASIC and the crust type to MEDIUM.

4. If the dough is too dense or too wet, adjust the amount of flour and liquid in the recipe.

5. When the program has ended, take the pan out of the bread machine and let cool for 5 minutes.

6. Shake the loaf out of the pan. If necessary, use a spatula.

7. Wrap the bread with a kitchen towel and set it aside for an hour. Otherwise, you can cool it on a wire rack.

Nutrition: Calories: 277 calories; Total Carbohydrate: 48.4 g Cholesterol: 9 g Total Fat: 4.7g Protein: 9.4 g Sodium: 547 mg Sugar: 3.3 g

Curvy Carrot Bread

Preparation Time: 2 hours

Cooking Time: 15 minutes

Servings: 12

Ingredients:

- ¾ cup milk, lukewarm

- tablespoons butter, melted at room temperature

- 1 tablespoon honey

- ¾ teaspoon ground nutmeg

- ½ teaspoon salt

- 1 ½ cups shredded carrot

- cups white bread flour

- ¼ teaspoons bread machine or active dry yeast

Directions:

1 Take 1 ½ pound size loaf pan and first add the liquid ingredients and then add the dry ingredients.

2 Place the loaf pan in the machine and close its top lid.

3   Plug the bread machine into power socket. For selecting a bread cycle, press "Quick Bread/Rapid Bread" and for selecting a crust type, press "Light" or "Medium".

4 Start the machine and it will start preparing the bread.

5 After the bread loaf is completed, open the lid and take out the loaf pan.

6 Allow the pan to cool down for 10-15 minutes on a wire rack. Gently shake the pan and remove the bread loaf.

7 Make slices and serve.

Nutrition: Calories: 142 calories; Total Carbohydrate: 32.2 g Cholesterol: 0 g Total Fat: 0.8 g Protein: 2.33 g

Potato Rosemary Bread

Preparation Time: 3 hours

Cooking Time: 30 minutes

Servings: 20

Ingredients:

- cups bread flour, sifted
- 1 tablespoon white sugar
- 1 tablespoon sunflower oil
- 1½ teaspoons salt
- 1½ cups lukewarm water
- 1 teaspoon active dry yeast
- 1 cup potatoes, mashed
- teaspoons crushed rosemary

Directions:

1 Prepare all of the ingredients for your bread and measuring means (a cup, a spoon, kitchen scales).

2 Carefully measure the ingredients into the pan, except the potato and rosemary.

3 Place all of the ingredients into the bread bucket in the right order, following the manual for your bread machine.

4 Close the cover.

5 Select the program of your bread machine to BREAD with FILLINGS and choose the crust color to MEDIUM.

6 Press START.

7 After the signal, put the mashed potato and rosemary to the dough.

8 Wait until the program completes.

9 When done, take the bucket out and let it cool for 5-10 minutes.

10 Shake the loaf from the pan and let cool for 30 minutes on a cooling rack.

11 Slice, serve and enjoy the taste of fragrant homemade bread.

Nutrition: Calories: 106 calories; Total Carbohydrate: 21 g Total Fat: 1 g Protein: 2.9 g Sodium: 641 mg Fiber: 1 g Sugar: 0.8 g

Beetroot Prune Bread

Preparation Time: 3 hours

Cooking Time: 30 minutes

Servings: 20

Ingredients:

- 1½ cups lukewarm beet broth
- 5¼ cups all-purpose flour
- 1 cup beet puree
- 1 cup prunes, chopped
- tablespoons extra virgin olive oil
- tablespoons dry cream
- 1 tablespoon brown sugar
- teaspoons active dry yeast
- 1 tablespoon whole milk
- teaspoons sea salt

Directions:

1 Prepare all of the ingredients for your bread and measuring means (a cup, a spoon, kitchen scales).

2 Carefully measure the ingredients into the pan, except the prunes.

3   Place all of the ingredients into the bread bucket in the right order, following the manual for your bread machine.

4 Close the cover.

5 Select the program of your bread machine to BASIC and choose the crust color to MEDIUM.

6 Press START.

7 After the signal, put the prunes to the dough.

8 Wait until the program completes.

9 When done, take the bucket out and let it cool for 5-10 minutes.

10   Shake the loaf from the pan and let cool for 30 minutes on a cooling rack.

11 Slice, serve and enjoy the taste of fragrant homemade bread.

Nutrition: Calories: 443 calories; Total Carbohydrate: 81.1 g Total Fat: 8.2 g Protein: 9.9 g Sodium: 604 mg Fiber: 4.4 g Sugar: 11.7 g

Black-Eyed Peas and Corn Salad

Preparation Time: 30 minutes

Cooking Time: 50 minutes

Servings: 4

Ingredients:

- 2½ cups cooked black-eyed peas
- 3 ears corn, kernels removed
- 1 medium ripe tomato, diced
- ½ medium red onion, peeled and diced small
- ½ red bell pepper, deseeded and diced small
- 1 jalapeño pepper, deseeded and minced
- ½ cup finely chopped cilantro
- ¼ cup plus 2 tablespoons balsamic vinegar
- 3 cloves garlic, peeled and minced
- 1 teaspoon toasted and ground cumin seeds

Directions:

1. Stir together all the ingredients in a large bowl and refrigerate for about 1 hour, or until well chilled.
2. Serve chilled.

Nutrition: Calories: 247 Fat: 1.8g Carbs: 47.6g Protein: 12.9g Fiber: 11.7g

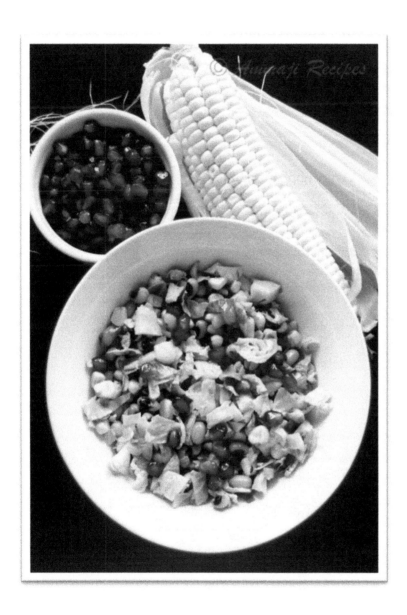

Walnut, Coconut, and Oat Granola

Preparation Time: 15 minutes

Cooking Time: 1 hour 40 minutes

Servings: 4

Ingredients:

- 1 cup chopped walnuts

- 1 cup unsweetened, shredded coconut

- 2 cups rolled oats

- 1 teaspoon ground cinnamon

- 2 tablespoons hemp seeds

- 2 tablespoons ground flaxseeds

- 2 tablespoons chia seeds

- ¾ teaspoon salt (optional)

- ¼ cup maple syrup

- ¼ cup water

- 1 teaspoon vanilla extract

- ½ cup dried cranberries

Directions:

1. Preheat the oven to 250°F (120°C). Line a baking sheet with parchment paper.

2. Mix the walnuts, coconut, rolled oats, cinnamon, hemp seeds, flaxseeds, chia seeds, and salt (if desired) in a bowl.

3. Combine the maple syrup and water in a saucepan. Bring to a boil over medium heat, then pour in the bowl of walnut mixture.

4. Add the vanilla extract to the bowl of mixture. Stir to mix well. Pour the mixture in the baking sheet, then level with a spatula so the mixture coat the bottom evenly.

5. Place the baking sheet in the preheated oven and bake for 90 minutes or until browned and crispy. Stir the mixture every 15 minutes.

6. Remove the baking sheet from the oven. Allow to cool for 10 minutes, then serve with dried cranberries on top.

Nutrition: Calories: 1870 Fat: 115.8g Carbs: 238.0g Protein: 59.8g Fiber: 68.9g

Chocó Chia Pudding

Preparation Time: 10 minutes

Cooking Time: 0 minutes

Servings: 6

Ingredients:

- 2 1/2 cups coconut milk

- 2 scoops stevia extract powder

- 6 tbsp. cocoa powder

- 1/2 cup chia seeds

- 1/2 tsp vanilla extract

- 1/8 cup xylitol

- 1/8 tsp salt

Directions:

1. Add all ingredients into the blender and blend until smooth.

2. Pour mixture into the glass container and place in refrigerator.

3. Serve chilled and enjoy.

Nutrition: Calories: 178 Total Carbohydrate: 3 g Cholesterol: 3 mg
Total Fat: 17 g Fiber: g Protein: 9 g Sodium: 297 mg

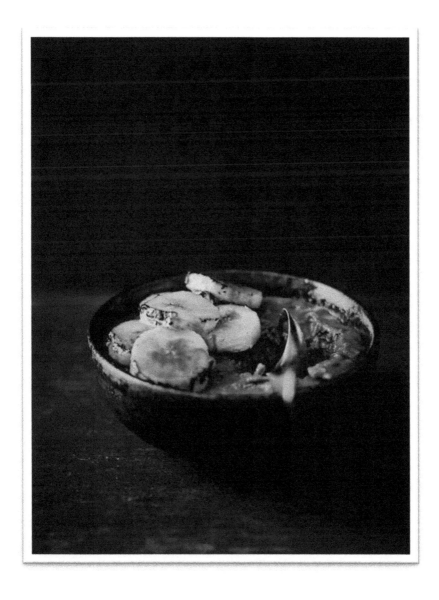

Spiced Buttermilk

Preparation Time: 5 minutes

Cooking Time: 0 minute

Servings: 2

Ingredients:

- 3/4 teaspoon ground cumin

- 1/4 teaspoon sea salt

- 1/8 teaspoon ground black pepper

- 2 mint leaves

- 1/8 teaspoon lemon juice

- ¼ cup cilantro leaves

- 1 cup of chilled water

- 1 cup vegan yogurt, unsweetened

- Ice as needed

Directions:

1. Place all the ingredients in the order in a food processor or blender, except for cilantro and ¼ teaspoon cumin, and then pulse for 2 to 3 minutes at high speed until smooth.

2. Pour the milk into glasses, top with cilantro and cumin, and then serve.

Nutrition: Calories: 211 Total Carbohydrate: 7 g Cholesterol: 13 mg Total Fat: 18 g Fiber: 3 g Protein: 17 g Sodium: 289 mg

Soothing Ginger Tea Drink

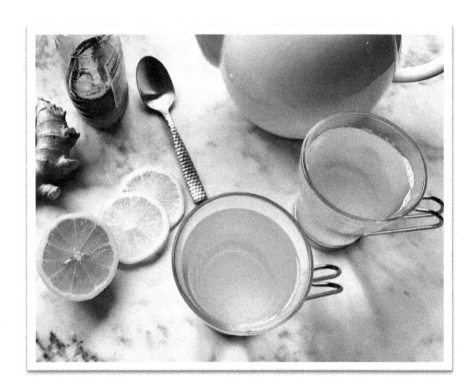

Preparation Time: 5 minutes

Cooking Time: 2 hours 20 minutes

Servings: 8

Ingredients:

- 1 tablespoon of minced gingerroot

- 2 tablespoons of honey

- 15 green tea bags

- 32 fluid ounce of white grape juice

- 2 quarts of boiling water

Directions:

1. Pour water into a 4-quarts slow cooker, immerse tea bags, cover the cooker and let stand for 10 minutes.

2. After 10 minutes, remove and discard tea bags and stir in remaining ingredients.

3. Return cover to slow cooker, then plug in and let cook at high heat setting for 2 hours or until heated through.

4. When done, strain the liquid and serve hot or cold.

Nutrition: Calories 232 Carbs: 7.9g Protein: 15.9g Fat: 15.1g

Nice Spiced Cherry Cider

Preparation Time: 1 hour 5 minutes

Cooking Time: 3 hours

Servings: 16

Ingredients:

- 2 cinnamon sticks, each about 3 inches long

- 6-ounce of cherry gelatin

- 4 quarts of apple cider

Directions:

1. Using a 6-quarts slow cooker, pour the apple cider and add the cinnamon stick.

2. Stir, then cover the slow cooker with its lid. Plug in the cooker and let it cook for 3 hours at the high heat setting or until it is heated thoroughly.

3. Then add and stir the gelatin properly, then continue cooking for another hour.

4. When done, remove the cinnamon sticks and serve the drink hot or cold.

Nutrition: Calories 78 Carbs: 13.2g Protein: 2.8g Fat: 1.5g

Peach-Mango Crumble (Pressure cooker)

Preparation Time: 10 minutes

Cooking Time: 6 minutes

Servings: 4-6

Ingredient:

- 3 cups chopped fresh or frozen peaches

- 3 cups chopped fresh or frozen mangos

- 4 tablespoons unrefined sugar or pure maple syrup, divided

- 1 cup gluten-free rolled oats

- ½ cup shredded coconut, sweetened or unsweetened

- 2 tablespoons coconut oil or vegan margarine

Directions:

1. Preparing the Ingredients. In a 6- to 7-inch round baking dish, toss together the peaches, mangos, and 2 tablespoons of sugar. In a food processor, combine the oats, coconut, coconut oil, and remaining 2 tablespoons of sugar. Pulse until combined. (If you use maple syrup, you'll need less coconut oil. Start with just the syrup and add oil if the

mixture isn't sticking together.) Sprinkle the oat mixture over the fruit mixture.

2. Cover the dish with aluminum foil. Put a trivet in the bottom of your electric pressure cooker's cooking pot and pour in a cup or two of water. Using a foil sling or silicone helper handles, lower the pan onto the trivet.

3. High pressure for 6 minutes. Close and lock the lid, and select High Pressure for 6 minutes.

4. Pressure Release. Once the Cooking Time: is complete, quick release the pressure. Unlock and remove the lid.

5. Let cool for a few minutes before carefully lifting out the dish with oven mitts or tongs. Scoop out portions to serve.

Nutrition: Calories 275 Fat 19 g Carbohydrates 19 g Sugar 4 g Protein 14 g Cholesterol 60 mg

Almond-Date Energy Bites

Preparation Time: 5 minutes

Cooking Time: 15 minutes

Servings: 24

Ingredients:

- 1 cup dates, pitted

- 1 cup unsweetened shredded coconut

- ¼ cup chia seeds

- ¾ cup ground almonds

- ¼ cup cocoa nibs, or non-dairy chocolate chips

Directions:

1. Purée everything in a food processor until crumbly and sticking together, pushing down the sides whenever necessary to keep it blending. If you don't have a food processor, you can mash soft Medjool dates. But if you're using harder baking dates, you'll have to soak them and then try to purée them in a blender.

2. Form the mix into 24 balls and place them on a baking sheet lined with parchment or waxed paper. Put in the fridge to set for about 15 minutes. Use the softest dates you can find. Medjool dates are the best for this purpose. The hard dates you see in the baking aisle of your supermarket are going to take a long time to blend up. If you use

those, try soaking them in water for at least an hour before you start, and then draining.

Nutrition: Calories 171 Fat 4 g Carbohydrates 7 g Sugar 7 g Protein 22 g Cholesterol 65 mg

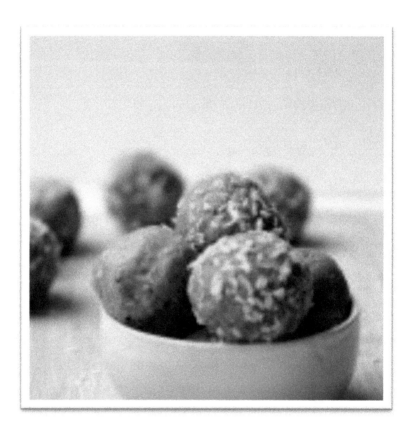

Pumpkin Pie Cups
(Pressure cooker)

Preparation Time: 5 minutes

Cooking Time: 6 minutes

Servings: 4-6

Ingredients:

- 1 cup canned pumpkin purée

- 1 cup nondairy milk

- 6 tablespoons unrefined sugar or pure maple syrup (less if using sweetened milk), plus more for sprinkling

- ¼ cup spelt flour or whole-grain flour

- ½ teaspoon pumpkin pie spice

- Pinch salt

Directions:

1. Preparing the Ingredients. In a medium bowl, stir together the pumpkin, milk, sugar, flour, pumpkin pie spice, and salt. Pour the mixture into 4 heat-proof ramekins. Sprinkle a bit more sugar on the top of each, if you like. Put a trivet in the bottom of your electric pressure cooker's cooking pot and pour in a cup or two of water. Place

the ramekins onto the trivet, stacking them if needed (3 on the bottom, 1 on top).

2. High pressure for 6 minutes. Close and lock the lid, and select High Pressure for 6 minutes.

3. Pressure Release. Once the Cooking Time: is complete, quick release the pressure. Unlock and remove the lid. Let cool for a few minutes before carefully lifting out the ramekins with oven mitts or tongs. Let cool for at least 10 minutes before serving.

Nutrition: Calories 152 Fat 4 g Carbohydrates 4 g Sugar 8 g Protein 18 g Cholesterol 51 mg

Fudgy Brownies
(Pressure cooker)

Preparation Time: 10 minutes

Cooking Time: 5 minutes

Servings: 4-6

Ingredients:

- 3 ounces dairy-free dark chocolate

- 1 tablespoon coconut oil or vegan margarine

- ½ cup applesauce

- 2 tablespoons unrefined sugar

- 1/3 cup whole-grain flour

- ½ teaspoon baking powder

- Pinch salt

Directions:

1. Preparing the Ingredients. Put a trivet in your electric pressure cooker's cooking pot and pour in a cup or two of two of water. Select Sauté or Simmer. In a large heat-proof glass or ceramic bowl, combine the chocolate and coconut oil. Place the bowl over the top of your

pressure cooker, as you would a double boiler. Stir occasionally until the chocolate is melted, then turn off the pressure cooker. Stir the applesauce and sugar into the chocolate mixture. Add the flour, baking powder, and salt and stir just until combined. Pour the batter into 3 heat-proof ramekins. Put them in a heat-proof dish and cover with aluminum foil. Using a foil sling or silicone helper handles, lower the dish onto the trivet. (Alternately, cover each ramekin with foil and place them directly on the trivet, without the dish.)

2. High pressure for 6 minutes. Close and lock the lid, and select High Pressure for 5 minutes.

3. Pressure Release. Once the Cooking Time: is complete, quick release the pressure. Unlock and remove the lid.

4. Let cool for a few minutes before carefully lifting out the dish, or ramekins, with oven mitts or tongs. Let cool for a few minutes more before serving.

5. Top with fresh raspberries and an extra drizzle of melted chocolate.

Nutrition: Calories 256 Fat 29 g Carbohydrates 1 g Sugar 0.5 g Protein 11 g Cholesterol 84 mg

Chocolate Macaroons

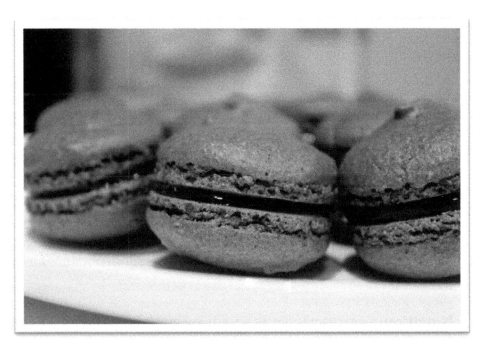

Preparation Time: 10 minutes

Cooking Time: 15 minutes

Servings: 8

Ingredients:

- 1 cup unsweetened shredded coconut

- 2 tablespoons cocoa powder

- 2/3 cup coconut milk

- ¼ cup agave

- pinch of sea salt

Directions:

1. Preparing the Ingredients.

2. Preheat the oven to 350°F. Line a baking sheet with parchment paper. In a medium saucepan, cook all the ingredients over -medium-high heat until a firm dough is formed. Scoop the dough into balls and place on the baking sheet.

3. Bake for 15 minutes, remove from the oven, and let cool on the baking sheet.

4. Serve cooled macaroons or store in a tightly sealed container for up to

Nutrition: Calories 371 Fat 15 g Carbohydrates 7 g Sugar 2 g Protein 41 g Cholesterol 135 mg

Express Coconut Flax Pudding

Preparation Time: 5 minutes

Cooking Time: 15 minutes

Servings: 4

Ingredients:

- 1 Tbsp. coconut oil softened

- 1 Tbsp. coconut cream

- 2 cups coconut milk canned

- 3/4 cup ground flax seed

- 4 Tbsp. coconut palm sugar (or to taste)

Directions:

1. Press SAUTÉ button on your Instant Pot

2. Add coconut oil, coconut cream, coconut milk, and ground flaxseed.

3. Stir about 5 - 10 minutes.

4. Lock lid into place and set on the MANUAL setting for 5 minutes.

5. When the timer beeps, press "Cancel" and carefully flip the Quick Release valve to let the pressure out.

6. Add the palm sugar and stir well.

7. Taste and adjust sugar to taste.

8. Allow pudding to cool down completely.

9. Place the pudding in an airtight container and refrigerate for up to 2 weeks.

Nutrition: Calories: 140 Fat: 2g Fiber: 23g Carbs: 22g Protein: 47g

Full-flavored Vanilla Ice Cream

Preparation Time: 5 minutes

Cooking Time: 20 minutes

Servings: 8

Ingredients:

- 1 1/2 cups canned coconut milk

- 1 cup coconut whipping cream

- 1 frozen banana cut into chunks

- 1 cup vanilla sugar

- 3 Tbsp. apple sauce

- 2 tsp pure vanilla extract

- 1 tsp Xanthan gum or agar-agar thickening agent

Directions:

1. Add all ingredients in a food processor; process until all ingredients combined well.

2. Place the ice cream mixture in a freezer-safe container with a lid over.

3. Freeze for at least 4 hours.

4. Remove frozen mixture to a bowl and beat with a mixer to break up the ice crystals.

5. Repeat this process 3 to 4 times.

6. Let the ice cream at room temperature for 15 minutes before serving.

Nutrition: Calories: 342 Fat: 15g Fiber: 11g Carbs: 8gProtein: 10g

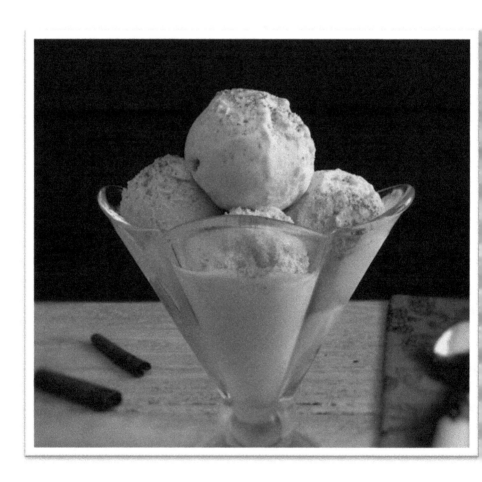

Crunchy Granola

Preparation Time: 10 Minutes

Cooking Time: 20 Minutes

Servings: 1

Ingredients:

- ½ cup Oats

- Dash of Salt

- 2 tbsp. Vegetable Oil

- 3 tbsp. Maple Syrup

- 1/3 cup Apple Cider Vinegar

- ½ cup Almonds

- 1 tsp. Cardamom, grounded

Directions:

1. Preheat the oven to 375 °F.

2. After that, mix oats, pistachios, salt, and cardamom in a large bowl.

3. Next, spoon in the vegetable oil and maple syrup to the mixture.

4. Then, transfer the mixture to a parchment-paper-lined baking sheet.

5. Bake them for 13 minutes or until the mixture is toasted. Tip: Check on them now and then. Spread it out well.

6. Return the sheet to the oven for further ten minutes.

7. From your oven remove the sheet and allow it to cool completely.

8. Serve and enjoy.

Nutrition: Calories: 763Kcal Proteins: 12.9g Carbohydrates: 64.8g Fat: 52.4g

Sweet Mango and Orange Dressing

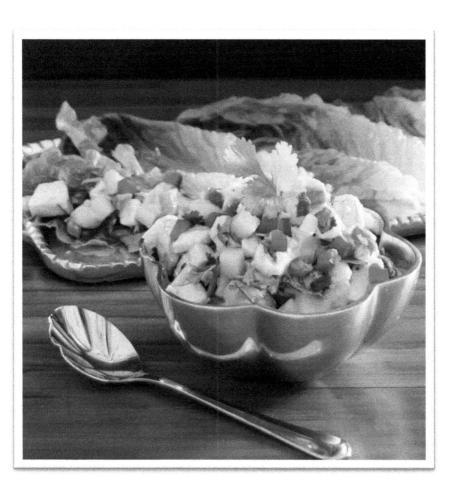

Preparation Time: 5 minutes

Cooking Time: 0 minutes

Servings: 1

Ingredients:

- 1 cup (165 g) diced mango, thawed if frozen

- ½ cup orange juice

- 2 tablespoons rice vinegar

- 2 tablespoons fresh lime juice

- ¼ teaspoon salt (optional)

- 1 teaspoon date sugar (optional)

- 2 tablespoons chopped cilantro

Directions:

1. Pulse all the ingredients except for the cilantro in a food processor until it reaches the consistency you like. Add the cilantro and whisk well.

2. Store in an airtight container in the fridge for up to 2 days.

Nutrition: Calories: 32 Fat: 0.1g Carbs: 7.4g Protein: 0.3g Fiber: 0.5g

Spinach & Dill Pasta Salad

Preparation Time: 5 minutes

Cooking Time: 0 minutes

Servings: 4

Ingredients:

For salad:

- 3 cups cooked whole-wheat fusilli

- 2 cups cherry tomatoes, halved

- ½ cup vegan cheese, shredded

- 4 cups spinach, chopped

- 2 cups edamame, thawed

- 1 large red onion, finely chopped

For dressing:

- 2 tablespoons white wine vinegar

- ½ teaspoon dried dill

- 2 tablespoons extra-virgin olive oil

- Salt to taste

- Pepper to taste

Directions:

To make dressing:

1. Add all the ingredients for dressing into a bowl and whisk well. Set aside for a while for the flavors to set in.

To make salad:

2. Add all the ingredients of the salad in a bowl. Toss well.

3. Drizzle dressing on top. Toss well.

4. Divide into 4 plates and serve.

Nutrition: Calories 684 Total Fat 33.6g Saturated Fat 4.6g Cholesterol 4mg Sodium 632mg Total Carbohydrate 69.5g Dietary Fiber 12g Total Sugars 6.4g Protein 31.7g Vitamin D 0mcg Calcium 368mg Iron 8mg Potassium 1241mg

Italian Veggie Salad

Preparation Time: 10 minutes

Cooking Time: 0 minutes

Servings: 8

Ingredients:

For salad:

- 1 cup fresh baby carrots, quartered lengthwise

- 1 celery rib, sliced

- 3 large mushrooms, thinly sliced

- 1 cup cauliflower florets, bite sized, blanched

- 1 cup broccoli florets, blanched

- 1 cup thinly sliced radish

- 4-5 ounces hearts of romaine salad mix to serve

For dressing:

- ½ package Italian salad dressing mix

- 3 tablespoons white vinegar

- 3 tablespoons water

- 3 tablespoons olive oil

- 3-4 pepperoncino, chopped

Directions:

To make salad:

1. Add all the ingredients of the salad except hearts of romaine to a bowl and toss.

To make dressing:

2. Add all the ingredients of the dressing in a small bowl. Whisk well.

3. Pour dressing over salad and toss well. Refrigerate for a couple of hours.

4. Place romaine in a large bowl. Place the chilled salad over it and serve.

Nutrition: Calories 84 Total Fat 6.7g Saturated Fat 1.2g Cholesterol 3mg Sodium 212mg Total Carbohydrate 5g Dietary Fiber 1.4g Total Sugars 1.6g Protein 2g Vitamin D 31mcg Calcium 27mg Iron 1mg Potassium 193mg

Honey Lime Quinoa Fruit Salad

Preparation Time: 20 Minutes

Cooking Time: 0 Minutes

Servings: 6

Ingredients:

- Basil, chopped, one tablespoon

- Lime juice, two tablespoons

- Mango, diced, one cup

- Blueberries, one cup

- Blackberries, one cup

- Strawberries, sliced, one and one half cup

- Quinoa, cooked, one cup

Directions:

1. In a large-sized bowl, mix the fruits with the cooked quinoa and mix well.

2. Drizzle on the lime juice and add the chopped basil and mix the fruit gently but thoroughly to coat all of the pieces.

Nutrition: Calories: 246 Protein: 7g Fat: 1g Carbs: 44g

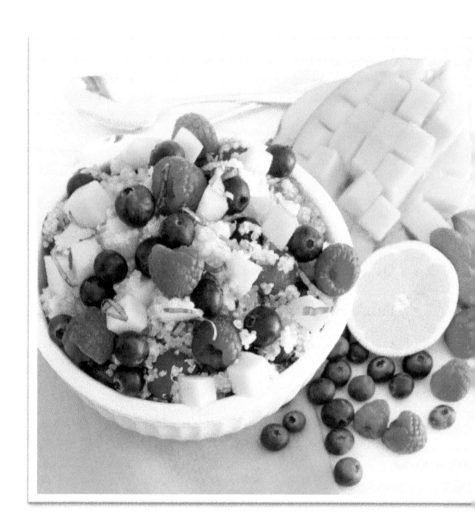

Sundried Tomato and Mushroom Penne Pasta

Preparation Time: 10 minutes

Cooking Time: 20 minutes

Servings: 4

Ingredients:

- Penne pasta, uncooked – 250 grams

- Corn starch – 2.5 tablespoons

- Olive oil – 4 teaspoons

- Garlic, minced – 6 cloves

- Sundried tomatoes, drained from the oil - .75 cup

- Soy milk (or almond), unsweetened – 2 cups

- Onion, diced – 1

- Oregano, dried -.5 teaspoon

- Nutritional yeast – 1 tablespoon

- Sea salt – 1 teaspoon

- Mushrooms, sliced – 1.5 cups

- Chili flakes – 1 teaspoon

- Black pepper, ground - .25 teaspoon

Directions:

1. Place the pasta in a large pot of salted boiling water and cook it according to the individual brand's instructions, but don't cook it quite all the way. Instead, allow the pasta to remain slightly under-cooked, as you will finish cooking it later on. Drain the pasta, reserving the pasta water.

2. Place a large frying pan on the large burner of your stove surface and set it to a medium temperature. Add in three teaspoons of the olive oil and the mushrooms, cooking for two minutes before adding in the garlic. Cook for an additional two minutes, until the mushrooms, are tender, and the garlic is fragrant.

3. Remove the mushrooms and garlic from the skillet and set them aside.

4. Add the corn starch, sea salt, and half of the soy milk into the hot skillet. Use a whisk to make sure that there are no clumps of corn starch and that the sauce is smooth. Once thickened, add the remaining soy milk and whisk again.

5. Into a blender pour the hot sauce mixture, nutritional yeast, half of the sundried tomatoes, and .33 cup of the hot pasta water. Blend the mixture on medium to high speed, being sure that it does not overflow from the heat buildup. Once blended smooth set the sauce aside.

6. Rinse out the previously used skillet and then add in the remaining teaspoon of olive oil. Chop the remaining sundried tomatoes and add them into the skillet along with the diced onion, allowing them to cook for three minutes until the onion becomes translucent. Add in the dried oregano and chili flakes, cooking the skillet for an additional minute until fragrant. If the ingredients begin to stick to the skillet simply add in a small amount of the reserved pasta water.

7. Add the prepared sauce into the skillet with the onion and sundried tomatoes, stirring all of the ingredients together. Add in the pasta, coating it in the sauce and adding any pasta water if you need to loosen the sauce.

8. Continue to cook the ingredients together until the pasta is al dente and then serve.

Nutrition: Number of Calories in Individual **Servings:** 350 Protein Grams: 14 Fat Grams: 8 Total Carbohydrates Grams: 55 Net Carbohydrates Grams: 50

Ritzy Fava Bean Ratatouille

Preparation Time: 15 minutes

Cooking Time: 40 minutes

Servings: 4

Ingredients:

- 1 medium red onion, peeled and thinly sliced

- 2 tablespoons low-sodium vegetable broth

- 1 large eggplant, stemmed and cut into ½-inch dice

- 1 red bell pepper, seeded and diced

- 2 cups cooked fava beans

- 2 Roma tomatoes, chopped

- 1 medium zucchini, diced

- 2 cloves garlic, peeled and finely chopped

- ¼ cup finely chopped basil

- Salt, to taste (optional)

- Ground black pepper, to taste

Directions:

1. Add the onion to a saucepan and sauté for 7 minutes or until caramelized.

2. Add the vegetable broth, eggplant and red bell pepper to the pan and sauté for 10 more minutes.

3. Add the fava beans, tomatoes, zucchini, and garlic to the pan and sauté for an additional 5 minutes.

4. Reduce the heat to medium-low. Put the pan lid on and cook for 15 minutes or until the vegetables are soft. Stir the vegetables halfway through.

5. Transfer them onto a large serving plate. Sprinkle with basil, salt (if desired), and black pepper before serving.

Nutrition: Calories: 114 Fat: 1.0g Carbs: 24.2g Protein: 7.4g Fiber: 10.3g

Lemon Mousse

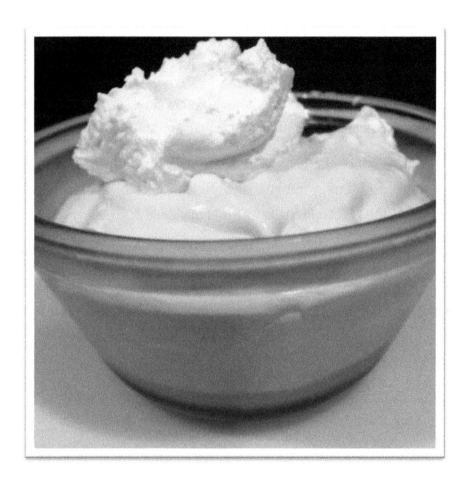

Preparation Time: 10 minutes

Cooking Time: 0 minute

Servings: 2

Ingredients:

- 14 oz. coconut milk
- 12 drops liquid stevia
- 1/2 tsp lemon extract
- 1/4 tsp turmeric

Directions:

1. Place coconut milk can in the refrigerator for overnight. Scoop out thick cream into a mixing bowl.

2. Add remaining ingredients to the bowl and whip using a hand mixer until smooth.

3. Transfer mousse mixture to a zip-lock bag and pipe into small serving glasses. Place in refrigerator.

4. Serve chilled and enjoy.

Nutrition: Calories: 189 Total Carbohydrate: 2 g Cholesterol: 13 mg Total Fat: 7 g Fiber: 2 g Protein: 15 g Sodium: 321 mg

Black-Eyed Pea, Beet, and Carrot Stew

Preparation Time: 15 minutes

Cooking Time: 40 minutes

Servings: 2

Ingredients:

- ½ cup black-eyed peas, soaked in water overnight
- 3 cups water
- 1 large beet, peeled and cut into ½-inch pieces (about ¾ cup)
- 1 large carrot, peeled and cut into ½-inch pieces (about ¾ cup)
- ¼ teaspoon turmeric
- ¼ teaspoon toasted and ground cumin seeds
- 1/8 teaspoon asafetida
- ¼ cup finely chopped parsley
- ¼ teaspoon cayenne pepper
- ¼ teaspoon salt (optional)
- ½ teaspoon fresh lime juice

Directions:

1. Pour the black-eyed peas and water in a pot, then cook over medium heat for 25 minutes.

2. Add the beet and carrot to the pot and cook for 10 more minutes. Add more water if necessary.

3. Add the turmeric, cumin, asafetida, parsley, and cayenne pepper to the pot and cook for an additional 6 minutes or until the vegetables are soft. Stir the mixture periodically. Sprinkle with salt, if desired.

4. Drizzle the lime juice on top before serving in a large bowl.

Nutrition: Calories: 84 | fat: 0.7g | carbs: 16.6g | protein: 4.1g | fiber: 4.5g

Koshari

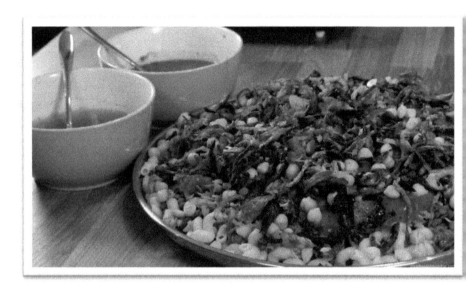

Preparation Time: 15 minutes

Cooking Time: 2 hours 10 minutes

Servings: 6

Ingredients:

- 1 cup green lentils, rinsed

- 3 cups water

- Salt, to taste (optional)

- 1 large onion, peeled and minced

- 2 tablespoons low-sodium vegetable broth

- 4 cloves garlic, peeled and minced

- ½ teaspoon ground allspice

- 1 teaspoon ground coriander

- 1 teaspoon ground cumin

- 2 tablespoons tomato paste

- ½ teaspoon crushed red pepper flakes

- 3 large tomatoes, diced

- 1 cup cooked medium-grain brown rice

- 1 cup whole-grain elbow macaroni, cooked, drained, and kept warm

- 1 tablespoon brown rice vinegar

Directions:

1. Put the lentils and water in a saucepan, and sprinkle with salt, if desired. Bring to a boil over high heat. Reduce the heat to medium, then put the pan lid on and cook for 45 minutes or until the water is mostly absorbed. Pour the cooked lentils in the bowl and set aside.

2. Add the onion to a nonstick skillet, then sauté over medium heat for 15 minutes or until caramelized.

3. Add vegetable broth and garlic to the skillet and sauté for 3 minutes or until fragrant.

4. Add the allspice, coriander, cumin, tomato paste, and red pepper flakes to the skillet and sauté for an additional 3 minutes until aromatic.

5. Add the tomatoes to the skillet and sauté for 15 minutes or until the tomatoes are wilted. Sprinkle with salt, if desired.

6. Arrange the cooked brown rice on the bottom of a large platter, then top the rice with macaroni, and then spread the lentils over. Pour the tomato mixture and brown rice vinegar over before serving.

Nutrition: Calories: 201 Fat: 1.6g Carbs: 41.8g Protein: 6.5g Fiber: 3.6g

Fragrant Spiced Coffee

Preparation Time: 10 minutes

Cooking Time: 3 hours

Servings: 8

Ingredients:

- 4 cinnamon sticks, each about 3 inches long

- 1 1/2 teaspoons of whole cloves

- 1/3 cup of honey

- 2-ounce of chocolate syrup

- 1/2 teaspoon of anise extract

- 8 cups of brewed coffee

Directions:

1. Pour the coffee in a 4-quarts slow cooker and pour in the remaining ingredients except for cinnamon and stir properly.

2. Wrap the whole cloves in cheesecloth and tie its corners with strings.

3. Immerse this cheesecloth bag in the liquid present in the slow cooker and cover it with the lid.

4. Then plug in the slow cooker and let it cook on the low heat setting for 3 hours or until heated thoroughly.

5. When done, discard the cheesecloth bag and serve.

Nutrition: Calories 136 Fat 12.6 g Carbohydrates 4.1 g Sugar 0.5 g Protein 10.3 g Cholesterol 88 mg

Inspirational Orange Smoothie

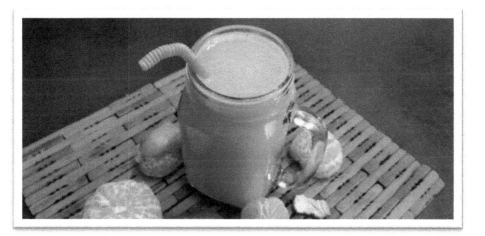

Preparation Time: 5 minutes

Cooking Time: 5 minutes

Servings: 1

Ingredients:

- 4 mandarin oranges, peeled

- 1 banana, sliced and frozen

- ½ cup non-fat Greek yoghurt

- ¼ cup coconut water

- 1 tsp vanilla extract

- 5 ice cubes

Directions:

1. Using a mixer, whisk all the ingredients.

2. Enjoy your drink!

Nutrition: Calories 256 Fat 13.3 g Carbohydrates 0 g Sugar 0 g Protein 34.5 g Cholesterol 78 mg

High Protein Blueberry Banana Smoothie

Preparation Time: 5 minutes

Cooking Time: 5 minutes

Servings: 2

Ingredients:

- 1 cup blueberries, frozen

- 2 ripe bananas

- 1 cup water

- 1 tsp vanilla extract

- 2 Tbsp. chia seeds

- ½ cup cottage cheese

- 1 tsp lemon zest

Directions:

1. Put all the smoothie ingredients into the blender and whisk until smooth.

2. Enjoy your wonderful smoothie!

Nutrition: Calories 358 Fat 19.8 g Carbohydrates 1.3 g Sugar 0.4 g Protein 41.9 g Cholesterol 131 mg

Ginger Smoothie with Citrus and Mint

Preparation Time: 5 minutes

Cooking Time: 3 minutes

Servings: 3

Ingredients:

- 1 head Romaine lettuce, chopped into 4 chunks

- 2 Tbsp. hemp seeds

- 5 mandarin oranges, peeled

- 1 banana, frozen

- 1 carrot

- 2-3 mint leaves

- ½ piece ginger root, peeled

- 1 cup water

- ¼ lemon, peeled

- ½ cup ice

Directions:

1.   Put all the smoothie ingredients in a blender and blend until smooth.

2. Enjoy!

Nutrition: Calories 101 Fat 4 g Carbohydrates 14 g Sugar 1 g Protein 2 g Cholesterol 3 mg

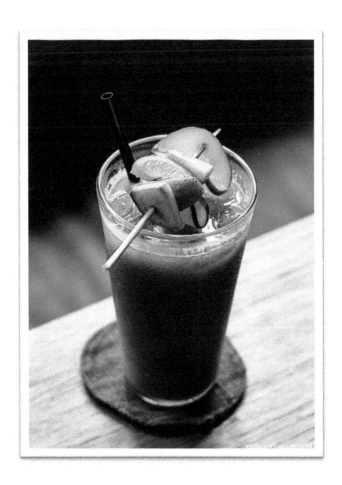

Strawberry Beet Smoothie

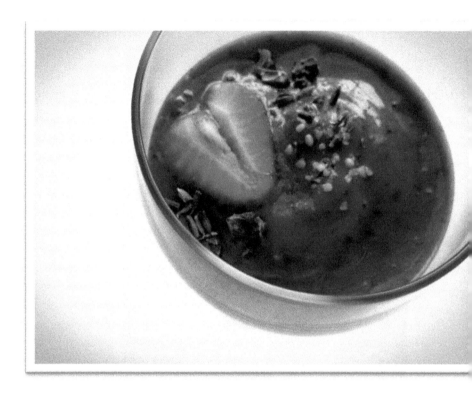

Preparation Time: 5 minutes

Cooking Time: 50 minutes

Servings: 2

Ingredients:

- 1 red beet, trimmed, peeled and chopped into cubes

- 1 cup strawberries, quartered

- 1 ripe banana

- ½ cup strawberry yoghurt

- 1 Tbsp. honey

- 1 Tbsp. water

- Milk, to taste

Directions:

1. Sprinkle the beet cubes with water, place on aluminum foil and put in the oven (preheated to 204°C). Bake for 40 minutes.

2. Let the baked beet cool.

3. Combine all the smoothie ingredients.

4. Enjoy your fantastic drink.

Nutrition: Calories 184 Fat 9.2 g Carbohydrates 1 g Sugar 0.4 g Protein 24.9 g Cholesterol 132 mg

Peanut Butter Shake

Preparation Time: 5 minutes

Cooking Time: 5 minutes

Servings: 2

Ingredients:

- 1 cup plant-based milk

- 1 handful kale

- 2 bananas, frozen

- 2 Tbsp. peanut butter

- ½ tsp ground cinnamon

- ¼ tsp vanilla powder

Directions:

1. Use a blender to combine all the ingredients for your shake.

2. Enjoy it!

Nutrition: Calories 184 Fat 9.2 g Carbohydrates 1 g Sugar 0.4 g Protein 24.9 g Cholesterol 132 mg

Strawberry Molasses Ice Cream

Preparation Time: 20 minutes

Cooking Time: 0 minute

Servings: 8

Ingredients:

- 1 lb. strawberries

- 3/4 cup coconut palm sugar (or granulated sugar)

- 1 cup coconut cream

- 1 Tbsp. molasses

- 1 tsp balsamic vinegar

- 1/2 tsp agar-agar

- 1/2 tsp pure strawberry extract

Directions:

1. Add strawberries, date sugar, and the balsamic vinegar in a blender; blend until completely combined.

2. Place the mixture in the refrigerator for one hour.

3. In a mixing bowl, beat the coconut cream with an electric mixer to make a thick mixture.

4. Add molasses, balsamic vinegar, agar-agar, and beat for further one minute or until combined well.

5. Keep frozen in a freezer-safe container (with plastic film and lid over).

Nutrition: Calories: 110 Fat: 31g Fiber: 18g Carbs: 15g Protein: 12g

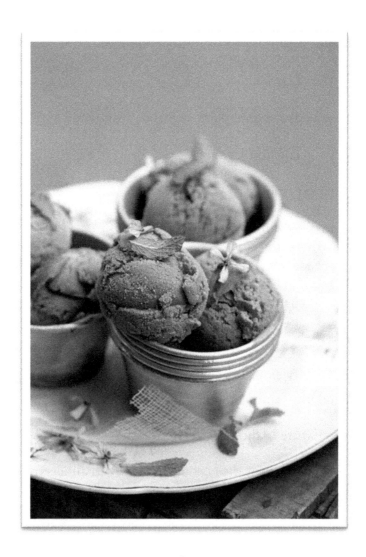

Strawberry-Mint Sorbet

Preparation Time: 10 minutes

Cooking Time: 5 minutes

Servings: 6

Ingredients:

- 1 cup of granulated sugar

- 1 cup of orange juice

- 1 lb. frozen strawberries

- 1 tsp pure peppermint extract

Directions:

1. Add sugar and orange juice in a saucepan.

2. Stir over high heat and boil for 5 minutes or until sugar dissolves.

3. Remove from the heat and let it cool down.

4. Add strawberries into a blender, and blend until smooth.

5. Pour syrup into strawberries, add peppermint extract and stir until all ingredients combined well.

6. Transfer mixture to a storage container, cover tightly, and freeze until ready to serve.

Nutrition: Calories: 257 Fat: 13g Fiber: 37g Carbs: 11g Protein: 8g

Keto Chocolate Brownies

Preparation Time: 15 minutes

Cooking Time: 15 minutes

Servings: 4

Ingredients:

- ¼ t. of the following:

- salt

- baking soda

- ½ c. of the following:

- sweetener of your choice

- coconut flour

- vegetable oil

- water

- ¼ c. of the following:

- cocoa powder

- almond milk yogurt

- 1 tbsp. ground flax

- 1 t. vanilla extract

Directions:

1. Bring the oven to 350 heat setting.

2. Mix the ground flax, vanilla, yogurt, oil, and water; set to the side for 10 minutes.

3. Line an oven-safe 8x8 baking dish with parchment paper.

4. After 10 minutes have passed, add coconut flour, cocoa powder, sweetener, baking soda, and salt.

5. Bake for 15 minutes; make sure that you placed it in the center. When they come out, they will look underdone.

6. Place in the refrigerator and let them firm up overnight.

Nutrition: Calories: 208 Fat: 3g Fiber: 4g Carbs: 7g Protein: 27g

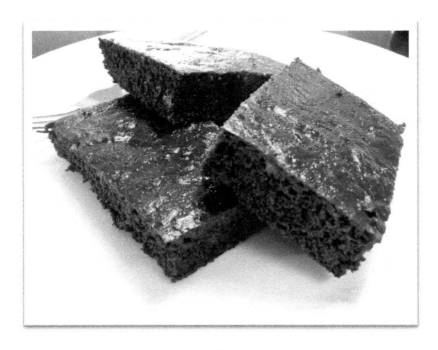

Chocolate Fat Bomb

Preparation Time: 5 minutes

Cooking Time: 0 minutes

Servings: 14

Ingredients:

- 1 tbsp. liquid sweetener of your choice.

- ¼ c. of the following:

- coconut oil, melted

- cocoa powder

- ½ c. almond butter

Directions:

1. Mix the ingredients in a medium bowl until smooth. Pour into the candy molds or ice cube trays.

2. Put in the freezer to set.

3. Store in freezer.

Nutrition: Calories: 241 Fat: 2g Fiber: 16g Carbs: 9g Protein: 22g

Chocolate Mousse

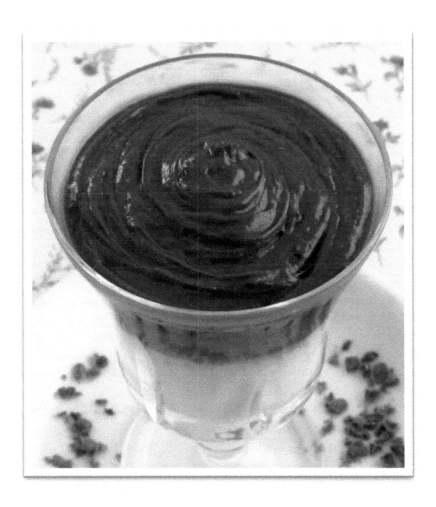

Preparation Time: 5 minutes

Cooking Time: 0 minute

Servings: 2

Ingredients:

- 6 drops liquid stevia extract

- ½ t. cinnamon

- 3 tbsp. cocoa powder, unsweetened

- 1 c. coconut milk

Directions:

1. On the day before, place the coconut milk into the refrigerator overnight.

2. Remove the coconut milk from the refrigerator; it should be very thick.

3. Whisk in cocoa powder with an electric mixer.

4. Add stevia and cinnamon and whip until combined.

5. Place in individual bowls and serve and enjoy.

Nutrition: Calories: 130 Fat: 5g Fiber: 3g Carbs: 6gProtein: 7g

Broccoli over Orzo

Preparation Time: 10 minutes

Cooking Time: 25 minutes

Servings: 3

Ingredients:

- 3 teaspoons olive oil

- 4 garlic cloves, smashed

- 2 cups broccoli florets

- 4½ ounces orzo pasta

- ¼ teaspoon salt

- ¼ teaspoon pepper

Directions:

1. Start off by preparing your broccoli. You can do this by trimming the stems off and slicing the broccoli into small, bite-size pieces. If you want, go ahead and season with salt.

2. Next, you will want to steam your broccoli over a little bit of water until it is cooked through. Once the broccoli is cooked, chop it up into even smaller pieces.

3. When the broccoli is done, cook your pasta according to the directions provided on the box. Once this is done, drain the water and then place the pasta back into the pot.

4. With the pasta and broccoli done, place it back into the pot with the garlic. Stir everything together well and cook until the garlic turns a nice golden colour. Be sure to stir everything to combine your meal well. Serve warm and enjoy a simple dinner!

Nutrition: Calories: 310 Fat: 4 g Carbs: 35 g Protein: 10 g

Sriracha Sauce

Preparation Time: 20 minutes

Cooking Time: 10 minutes

Servings: 2

Ingredients

- 15 red Fresno chilies, chopped into chunks

- ½ tablespoon salt

- 4 garlic cloves

- ¼ cup apple cider or white vinegar

- 2 tablespoons raw sugar

Directions:

1. Place the chilies, garlic, salt and sugar into a food processor. Pulse until coarsely chopped. Transfer into a mason's jar.

2. Cover with a plastic cling and leave it for 5-7 days to ferment. Stir often during this period. In 3-4 days you will see some bubbles appearing.

3. Transfer the contents of the jar into a blender. Add vinegar and blend until smooth.

4. Transfer into a saucepan after passing through a wire mesh strainer.

5. Bring to a boil on high heat.

6. When it starts boiling, reduce the heat and simmer for 5 minutes. Remove from heat and cool.

7. Transfer into a flip top bottle. Refrigerate until use.

Nutrition: Calories: 90 Fat: 6 g Carbs: 5 g Protein: 1 g

Potato Bread

Preparation Time: 3 hours

Cooking Time: 45 minutes

Servings: 2 loaves

Ingredients:

- 1 3/4 teaspoon active dry yeast
- tablespoon dry milk
- 1/4 cup instant potato flakes
- tablespoon sugar
- cups bread flour
- 1 1/4 teaspoon salt
- tablespoon butter
- 1 3/8 cups water

Directions:

1 Put all the liquid ingredients in the pan. Add all the dry ingredients, except the yeast. Form a shallow hole in the middle of the dry ingredients and place the yeast.

2 Secure the pan in the machine and close the lid. Choose the basic setting and your desired color of the crust. Press starts.

3 Allow the bread to cool before slicing.

Nutrition: Calories: 35calories; Total Carbohydrate: 19 g Total Fat: 0 g Protein: 4 g

Onion Potato Bread

Preparation Time: 1 hour 20 minutes

Cooking Time: 45 minutes

Servings: 2 loaves

Ingredients:

- tablespoon quick rise yeast

- cups bread flour

- 1 1/2 teaspoon seasoned salt

- tablespoon sugar

- 2/3 cup baked potatoes, mashed

- 1 1/2 cup onions, minced

- large eggs

- tablespoon oil

- 3/4 cup hot water, with the temperature of 115 to 125 degrees F (46 to 51 degrees C)

Directions:

1   Put the liquid ingredients in the pan. Add the dry ingredients, except the yeast. Form a shallow well in the middle using your hand and put the yeast.

2 Place the pan in the machine, close the lid and turn it on. Select the express bake 80 setting and start the machine.

3 Once the bread is cooked, leave on a wire rack for 20 minutes or until cooled.

Nutrition: Calories: 160calories; Total Carbohydrate: 44 g Total Fat: 2 g Protein: 6 g

Spinach Bread

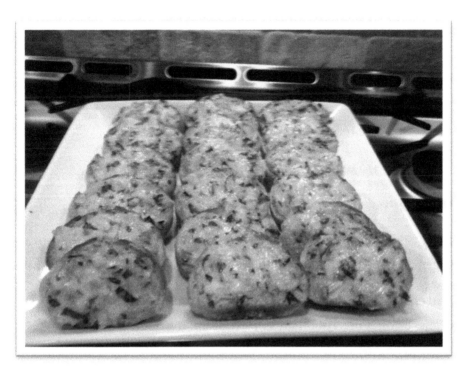

Preparation Time: 2 hours 20 minutes

Cooking Time: 40 minutes

Servings: 1 loaf

Ingredients:

- 1 cup water

- 1 tablespoon vegetable oil

- 1/2 cup frozen chopped spinach, thawed and drained

- cups all-purpose flour

- 1/2 cup shredded Cheddar cheese

- 1 teaspoon salt

- 1 tablespoon white sugar

- 1/2 teaspoon ground black pepper

- 1/2 teaspoons active dry yeast

Directions:

1   In the pan of bread machine, put all ingredients according to the suggested order of manufacture. Set white bread cycle.

Nutrition: Calories: 121 calories; Total Carbohydrate: 20.5 g Cholesterol: 4 mg Total Fat: 2.5 g Protein: 4 g Sodium: 184 mg

Easy Lemon Tahini Dressing

Preparation Time: 5 minutes

Cooking Time: 0 minutes

Servings: 1

Ingredients:

- ½ cup tahini

- ¼ cup fresh lemon juice (about 2 lemons)

- 1 teaspoon maple syrup

- 1 small garlic clove, chopped

- 1/8 teaspoon black pepper

- ¼ teaspoon salt (optional)

- ¼ to ½ cup water

Directions:

1. Process the tahini, lemon juice, maple syrup, garlic, black pepper, and salt (if desired) in a blender (high-speed blenders work best for this). Gradually add the water until the mixture is completely smooth.

2. Store in an airtight container in the fridge for up to 5 days.

Nutrition: Calories: 128 Fat: 9.6g Carbs: 6.8g Protein: 3.6g Fiber: 1.9

Edamame & Ginger Citrus Salad

Preparation Time: 15 minutes

Cooking Time: 0 minutes

Servings: 3

Ingredients:

Dressing:

- ¼ cup orange juice

- 1 tsp. lime juice

- ½ tbsp. maple syrup

- ½ tsp. ginger, finely minced

- ½ tbsp. sesame oil

Salad:

- ½ cup dry green lentils

- 2 cups carrots, shredded

- 4 cups kale, fresh or frozen, chopped

- 1 cup edamame, shelled

- 1 tablespoon roasted sesame seeds

- 2 tsp. mint, chopped

- Salt and pepper to taste

- 1 small avocado, peeled, pitted, diced

Directions:

1. Prepare the lentils according to the method.

2. Combine the orange and lime juices, maple syrup, and ginger in a small bowl. Mix with a whisk while slowly adding the sesame oil.

3. Add the cooked lentils, carrots, kale, edamame, sesame seeds, and mint to a large bowl.

4. Add the dressing and stir well until all the ingredients are coated evenly.

5. Store or serve topped with avocado and an additional sprinkle of mint.

Nutrition: Calories 507 Total Fat 23.1g Saturated Fat 4g Cholesterol 0mg Sodium 303mg Total Carbohydrate 56.8g Dietary Fiber 21.6g Total Sugars 8.4g Protein 24.6g Vitamin D 0mcg Calcium 374mg Iron 8mg Potassium 1911mg

Chickpea and Spinach Salad

Preparation Time: 5 minutes

Cooking Time: 0 minutes

Servings: 4

Ingredients:

- 2 cans (14.5 ounces each) chickpeas, drained, rinsed
- 7 ounces vegan feta cheese, crumbled or chopped
- 1 tablespoon lemon juice
- 1/3 -½ cup olive oil
- ½ teaspoon salt or to taste
- 4-6 cups spinach, torn
- ½ cup raisins
- 2 tablespoons honey
- 1-2 teaspoons ground cumin
- 1 teaspoon chili flakes

Directions:

1. Add cheese, chickpeas and spinach into a large bowl.
2. To make dressing: Add rest of the ingredients into another bowl and mix well.

3. Pour dressing over the salad. Toss well and serve.

Nutrition: Calories 822 Total Fat 42.5g Saturated Fat 11.7g Cholesterol 44mg Sodium 910mg Total Carbohydrate 89.6g Dietary Fiber 19.7g Total Sugars 32.7g Protein 29g Vitamin D 0mcg Calcium 417mg Iron 9mg Potassium 1347mg

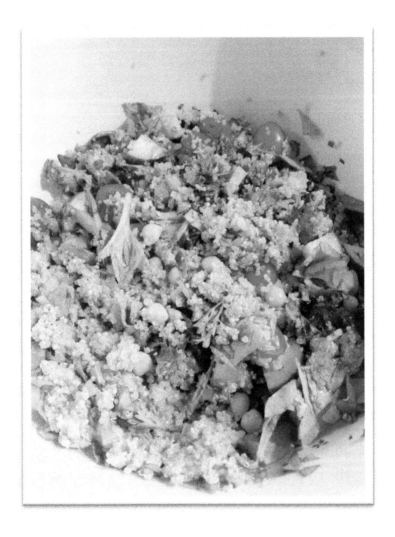

Mimosa Salad

Preparation Time: 10 Minutes

Cooking Time: 0 Minutes

Servings: 8

Ingredients:

- Mint, fresh, one half cup

- Orange juice, one half cup

- Pineapple, one cup cut into small pieces

- Strawberries, one cup cut into quarters

- Blueberries, one cup

- Blackberries, one cup

- Kiwi, three peeled and sliced

Directions:

1. In a large-sized bowl, mix all of the fruits together and then top with the orange juice and the fresh mint.

2. Toss gently together all of the fruit until they are well mixed.

Nutrition: Calories: 215 Protein: 3g Fat: 1g Carbs: 49g

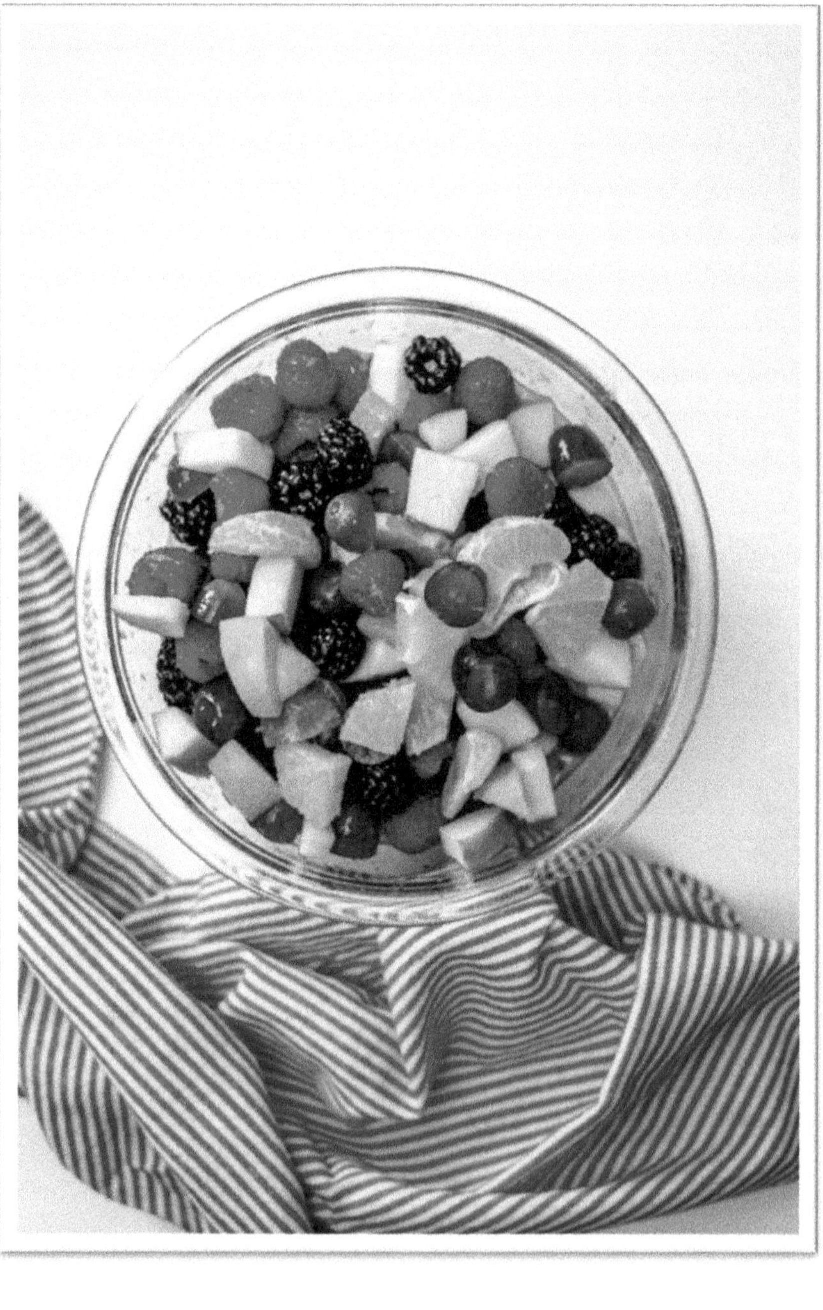

Lightning Source UK Ltd.
Milton Keynes UK
UKHW020635220621
385949UK00001B/53